MIND over MATTERS

I0479255

"A Guild to managing mental health"

The Healing and Hope Process

Hary Wins

Table of Content

Introduction:

21.

22.

23.

Introduction

Welcome to 'Mind Over Matter: A Guide to Managing Mental Health.' This book is designed to provide you with the knowledge, tools, and resources to take control of your mental health and well-being.

Mental health is an important and often overlooked aspect of our overall well-being. Many of us struggle with mental health issues at some point in our lives, yet we often feel alone, lost, and without guidance on how to handle it.

This book is here to change that. It is written in an engaging, friendly, and relatable tone, and is packed with practical advice, tips, and strategies to help you understand, manage and overcome mental health challenges.

We will explore the different types of mental health issues, their causes and triggers, and the available treatments and support options. You will learn about the importance of self-care, mindfulness, and positive thinking, and gain an understanding of how to navigate the mental health system.

But this book is not just about managing mental health challenges, it is also about thriving. It is an inspiration to you to understand that you are not alone and that you can overcome any mental health issue that you might be facing.

Throughout the book, you will find stories of people who have faced and overcome mental health challenges, and you will be inspired by their resilience and determination. You will also find practical exercises and worksheets to help you apply the strategies and techniques covered in the book to your own life.

So whether you are dealing with a mental health issue yourself, or you are looking to support someone you care about, 'Mind Over Matter' is your guide to managing and overcoming mental health challenges. It is time to take control of your mental health, and this book is here to help you do just that."

This book is also a guide to help you understand the importance of mental health in our lives, and how it affects all aspects of our lives. From our relationships, work, and daily routines, to our physical health and overall well-being, mental health plays a crucial role.

You will also learn about the different types of mental health conditions, such as anxiety, depression, bipolar disorder, and schizophrenia, and how to recognize the signs and symptoms. We will also explore the various treatment options available, including therapy, medication, and alternative therapies. We will also talk about the importance of seeking help and support, and how to find the right professional for you.

In addition, this book will also help you understand how to create a healthy and supportive environment for yourself and those around you. We will cover topics such as building a support network, how to talk about mental health, and how to advocate for mental health in your community.

Throughout the book, you will also find tips and strategies to help you maintain good mental health, such as how to practice self-care, how to manage stress, and how to develop a positive mindset. We will also discuss the importance of setting boundaries, managing your time, and finding balance in your life.

In 'Mind Over Matter,' we will take a holistic approach to mental health, looking at the whole person, not just the condition. This book is for everyone, whether you are dealing with a mental health issue or looking to support a loved one. It is a guide to understanding, managing, and overcoming mental health challenges, and to living a fulfilling and meaningful life.

Chapter 1

UNDERSTANDING MENTAL HEALTH

Mental health is an essential aspect of our overall well-being, influencing how we think, feel, and behave. It affects our relationships, work, and daily routines, and also plays a crucial role in our physical health. However, despite its importance, mental health is often overlooked and misunderstood. In this chapter, we will explore the basics of mental health, including what it is, why it matters, and the different factors that can impact it.

What is Mental Health? Mental health refers to our emotional, psychological, and social well-being. It affects how we think, feels, and behave in our daily lives. Good mental health allows us to cope with the stresses of life, work productively, and make meaningful contributions to our communities. On the other hand, poor mental health can lead to a range of problems, including difficulty in relationships, work, and daily routines, and can also affect our physical health.

Why Mental Health Matters Mental health matters because it affects all aspects of our lives. It influences how we think, feel, and behave, and also plays a crucial role in our physical health. Poor mental health can lead to a range of problems, including difficulty in relationships, work, and daily routines, and can also affect our physical health.

Factors that Impact Mental Health Mental health is influenced by a range of factors, including our genetics, environment, and lifestyle. Our biology, including the functioning of our brain and hormones, also plays a role. Additionally, social determinants of health, such as poverty, discrimination, and lack of access to education and resources, can also impact mental health. We have explored the basics of mental health, including what it is, why it matters, and the different factors that can impact it. Understanding mental health is the first step in managing and maintaining good mental health. In the following chapters, we will dive deeper into the different types of mental health conditions, the causes and triggers of mental health issues, and the various treatment options available. We will also explore how to create a healthy and supportive environment for yourself and those around you, and how to maintain good mental health. In addition to the factors already mentioned, other factors that can impact mental health include:

- Trauma and abuse: Exposure to traumatic events or experiences, such as physical, emotional, or sexual abuse, can lead to mental health issues such as PTSD (post-traumatic stress disorder).
- Loss and grief: The loss of a loved one or a significant life change can lead to feelings of grief and depression.
- Life transitions: Major life changes, such as starting a new job, moving to a new place, or getting married, can be stressful and can impact mental health.
- Substance abuse: The use of drugs and alcohol can harm mental health and can lead to addiction and other mental health issues.
- Medical conditions: Chronic physical health conditions can lead to mental health issues such as depression and anxiety.

It's also important to note that mental health is not a binary state. It's not simply a case of being "mentally healthy" or "mentally ill." Mental health exists on a spectrum, and we all have moments when our mental health is better or worse. Furthermore, it's not uncommon for people to have multiple mental health conditions at the same time. Mental health is a vital aspect of our overall well-being.

It is influenced by a range of factors, including genetics, environment, lifestyle, and social determinants of health. It's essential to understand and acknowledge the impact of these factors on mental health, to create a supportive environment for ourselves and those around us, and to maintain good mental health. It's also important to note that mental health is not limited to the presence or absence of a mental illness. Mental health encompasses a wide range of aspects, including emotional well-being, cognitive functioning, and social functioning. Emotional well-being, for example, refers to the ability to experience positive emotions, such as happiness and contentment, as well as the ability to cope with negative emotions, such as stress and sadness. Cognitive functioning refers to the ability to think, reason, and remember. Social functioning refers to the ability to interact with others and participate in social activities. Maintaining good mental health means taking care of not only the presence or absence of mental illness but also these various aspects of mental health. It means developing healthy coping mechanisms, establishing positive relationships, and participating in activities that bring joy and fulfillment. It's also important to note that mental health is not something that can be achieved and then maintained indefinitely.

It's a continuous process, requiring ongoing effort and attention. Furthermore, it's not something that can be achieved alone. Support from friends, family and healthcare professionals is essential in maintaining good mental health. In conclusion, understanding mental health is essential for managing and maintaining good mental health. It is influenced by a range of factors, including genetics, environment, lifestyle, and social determinants of health. It encompasses emotional, cognitive, and social well-being and requires ongoing effort and attention. Good mental health is not a destination, but a continuous journey that requires the support of loved ones, and healthcare professionals.

Chapter 2

Recognizing the Signs and Symptoms of Mental Health Conditions

Recognizing the signs and symptoms of mental health conditions is an important step in seeking help and support. However, it's important to note that the signs and symptoms of mental health conditions can vary greatly from person to person and can also change over time. Additionally, some people may not experience any signs or symptoms at all.

That being said, there are some common signs and symptoms that can indicate the presence of a mental health condition. These include:

Persistent feelings of sadness, hopelessness, or helplessness
Loss of interest in activities that were once enjoyable
Difficulty concentrating or making decisions
Changes in appetite or sleep patterns
Irritability or restlessness
Fatigue or lack of energy
Thoughts of self-harm or suicide
Extreme mood swings or sudden changes in mood
Delusions or hallucinations

It's also important to note that some mental health conditions may have physical symptoms as well. For example, anxiety can cause physical symptoms such as sweating, rapid heartbeat, and muscle tension.

If you or someone you know is experiencing any of these signs or symptoms, it's important to seek help. A mental health professional, such as a psychiatrist, psychologist, or counselor, can help determine if a mental health condition is present and recommend appropriate treatment options. It's also important to note that seeking help and support is a sign of strength, not weakness. Mental health conditions are not a personal failure and are not something that can be simply "gotten over." With the right treatment and support, recovery is possible, and many people with mental health conditions lead fulfilling and productive lives.

It's also important to understand that some people may not want to seek help or may not be aware that they have a mental health condition. This is why it's important for family members, friends, and loved ones to be aware of the signs and symptoms of mental health conditions and to be supportive of those who may be struggling. If you notice that a loved one is experiencing signs or symptoms of a mental health condition, you can encourage them to seek help and offer to help them find resources. It's also important to recognize that some groups of people may be at a higher risk for certain mental health conditions. For example, people who have experienced trauma, such as veterans or survivors of abuse, may be at a higher risk for post-traumatic stress disorder (PTSD). People who have a family history of mental health conditions may also be at a higher risk. Understanding these risk factors can help people to be more aware of their mental health and to seek help if needed. It's also important to note that mental health conditions can co-occur with other health conditions. For example, people with depression may also have chronic health conditions such as diabetes or heart disease. It's important for healthcare providers to be aware of this and to work together to provide comprehensive care.

In addition, it's important to understand that mental health is not only about the absence of mental illness, but also about overall well-being and resilience. To promote mental health, it's important to focus on self-care and stress management, practice healthy habits, and seek support when needed.

In conclusion, recognizing the signs and symptoms of mental health conditions is an important step in seeking help and support. It's important for everyone to be aware of the signs and symptoms, and to be supportive of those who may be struggling. Some groups of people may be at a higher risk for certain mental health conditions, and it's important to understand that mental health conditions can co-occur with other health conditions. Additionally, mental health is not only about the absence of mental illness, but also about overall well-being and resilience.

Chapter 3

UNDERSTANDING THE DIFFERENT TYPES OF MENTAL HEALTH CONDITIONS

Mental health conditions are a diverse group of disorders that can affect a person's thoughts, emotions, and behavior. There are many different types of mental health conditions, each with its own set of signs and symptoms, causes, and treatments. Understanding the different types of mental health conditions can help individuals to better understand their own experiences and to seek appropriate help and support.

Some of the most common types of mental health conditions include:

1.   Anxiety disorders: Anxiety disorders are characterized by excessive worry, nervousness, and fear. Examples of anxiety disorders include generalized anxiety disorder, panic disorder, and phobias.
2.   Mood disorders: Mood disorders are characterized by persistent feelings of sadness,

hopelessness, or helplessness. Examples of mood disorders include depression and bipolar disorder..

3. Schizophrenia: Schizophrenia is a severe mental health condition that affects how a person thinks, feels, and behaves. It can cause hallucinations, delusions, and disordered thinking.
4. Eating disorders: Eating disorders are characterized by abnormal eating habits and preoccupation with food and weight. Examples of eating disorders include anorexia nervosa and bulimia nervosa.
5. Personality disorders: Personality disorders are characterized by long-term patterns of thoughts, feelings, and behaviors that deviate from cultural norms and cause distress or impairment. Examples of personality disorders include borderline personality disorder and narcissistic personality disorder.
6. Trauma-related disorders: Trauma-related disorders are characterized by symptoms that occur as a result of exposure to a traumatic event. Examples of trauma-related disorders include PTSD and complex post-traumatic stress disorder.

It's important to note that these are just a few examples of the many different types of mental health conditions that exist. Each condition is unique and can affect people differently. Additionally, some people may experience more than one mental health condition at the same time.

Mental health conditions are a diverse group of disorders that can affect a person's thoughts, emotions, and behavior. There are many different types of mental health conditions, each with its own set of signs and symptoms, causes, and treatments. Understanding the different types of mental health conditions can help individuals to better understand their own experiences and to seek appropriate help and support. Some of the common types of mental health conditions include anxiety disorders, mood disorders, schizophrenia, eating disorders, personality disorders, and trauma-related disorders.

It's also important to note that many people experience mental health conditions without even realizing it. They may think that their symptoms are just a normal part of life or that they can handle them on their own. This can lead to a delay in seeking help and treatment. It's crucial to be aware of the signs and symptoms of mental health conditions and to understand that seeking help is a sign of strength, not weakness.

In this chapter, we will delve deeper into the different types of mental health conditions and their respective signs and symptoms.

We will also discuss the causes and risk factors that contribute to the development of these conditions. Individuals need to have a better understanding of the different types of mental health conditions so that they can identify when they or someone they know may be struggling with one. Additionally, we will also touch on the impact of mental health conditions on the individual's overall well-being and how it can affect their daily lives. We will also discuss the importance of early identification and intervention, and the various treatment options available for mental health conditions. This chapter is designed to provide readers with a comprehensive understanding of the different types of mental health conditions, their signs, symptoms, causes, and treatment options. Individuals need to be informed and educated about mental health conditions so that they can better understand and support themselves and others who may be struggling with one.

In summary, this chapter provides a detailed overview of the different types of mental health conditions, their signs, symptoms, causes, and treatment options, as it also discusses the importance of early identification and intervention, and the impact of mental health conditions on the individual's overall well-being.

The goal of this chapter is to educate readers and increase their understanding of mental health conditions, so they can better support themselves and others who may be struggling with one.

Chapter 4

Understanding and Managing Stress and Its Impact on Mental Health

Stress is a natural part of life, but when it becomes chronic, it can have a significant impact on mental health. Chronic stress can lead to a wide range of mental health conditions, including anxiety, depression, and PTSD. It's important to understand and manage stress to protect and maintain mental health.

Stress can come from a variety of sources, including work, relationships, financial difficulties, and personal health issues. It's important to identify the sources of stress in one's life and to develop strategies for managing them.

One effective way of managing stress is through relaxation techniques such as deep breathing, meditation, and yoga. Exercise, a healthy diet, and getting enough sleep are also important for managing stress.

Another way to manage stress is by practicing good time management and setting realistic goals and boundaries. It's also important to develop a support system of friends, family, and professionals that can provide a sounding board and offer advice and guidance.

Another important aspect of managing stress is learning how to cope with difficult emotions, such as anger and sadness, healthily. This can include talking to a therapist, journaling, or engaging in creative outlets such as art or music.

It's also important to remember that stress is a normal part of life and it's okay to feel overwhelmed at times. It's important to give yourself permission to take a break and engage in self-care.

In this chapter, we will delve deeper into the causes and effects of stress on mental health, and discuss the various ways of managing stress. We will also discuss the importance of self-care and the role of support systems in managing stress.

This chapter is designed to provide readers with a comprehensive understanding of stress and its impact on mental health, as well as strategies for managing it. The goal of this chapter is to educate readers on the importance of stress management and to equip them with the tools they need to protect and maintain their mental health.

Causes and Triggers of Mental Health Issues

Mental health conditions, such as anxiety and depression, can be caused by a variety of factors. Understanding the causes and triggers of mental health issues is essential for effective treatment and management. In this chapter, we will explore the various causes and triggers of mental health issues, including biological, psychological, and environmental factors.

Biological Factors: Biological factors refer to the physical and genetic factors that can contribute to the development of mental health conditions. These can include changes in brain chemistry, hormonal imbalances, and genetic predispositions. For example, research has shown that individuals with a family history of mental health conditions are more likely to develop a mental health condition themselves.

Psychological Factors: Psychological factors refer to the cognitive and emotional factors that can contribute to the development of mental health conditions. These can include past traumatic experiences, negative thought patterns, and low self-esteem. For example, an individual who has experienced a traumatic event such as sexual or physical abuse may be at a higher risk of developing PTSD. An example would be Jane, who was sexually abused as a child. She has struggled with anxiety and depression for years and has found that even the smallest triggers such as a hug from a stranger can bring back the traumatic memories and make her feel anxious and depressed.

Environmental Factors: Environmental factors refer to the external factors that can contribute to the development of mental health conditions. These can include stress, social isolation, and exposure to violence or other traumatic events. For example, another example of this is John, who lives in a high-crime area and has to walk home alone at night. He struggles with anxiety and often finds himself feeling paranoid and anxious about his safety. He has found that he feels much better when he takes a different route home or has someone walk with him.

Some examples of triggers of mental health issues can be:

- A person who suffered from a traumatic experience like sexual or physical abuse can trigger PTSD symptoms when they are reminded of the event, such as watching a movie that has similar themes.
- A person with bipolar disorder may experience manic or depressive episodes as a result of changes in their sleep schedule, such as jet lag or shift work.
- A person with a social anxiety disorder may experience symptoms when they are in a social situation, such as meeting new people or speaking in public.

It's important to note that mental health conditions can be caused by a combination of factors and that different individuals may be affected differently. For example, two people with the same mental health condition may have very different triggers for their symptoms. In this chapter, we will delve deeper into the various causes and triggers of mental health issues and discuss how these factors can affect individuals differently. We will also provide real-life examples to help readers understand how these causes and triggers may manifest in different situations.

The goal of this chapter is to provide readers with a comprehensive understanding of the causes and triggers of mental health issues and to equip them with the knowledge they need to identify and manage these factors in their own lives.

In summary, chapter 4 will provide a detailed overview of the causes and triggers of mental health issues, including biological, psychological, and environmental factors. The chapter will also provide real-life examples to help readers understand how these causes and triggers may manifest in different situations. The goal of this chapter is to provide readers with a comprehensive understanding of the causes and triggers of mental health issues and to equip them with the knowledge they need to identify and manage these factors in their own lives.

Chapter 5

NAVIGATING THE MENTAL HEALTH SYSTEM: FINDING THE RIGHT HELP

Navigating the mental health system can be a daunting task, especially for those who are struggling with a mental health condition. It can be difficult to know where to turn for help, and even more challenging to find the right kind of help. This chapter will provide a comprehensive guide to finding the right mental health professionals and resources, with a focus on real-life examples and an entertaining tone.

First, it is important to understand the different types of mental health professionals. There are several types of therapists, including psychologists, psychiatrists, licensed clinical social workers, and licensed professional counselors. Each type of therapist has its own unique set of qualifications and expertise, so it is important to choose the right one for your specific needs.

For example, a psychologist typically has a Ph.D. or PsyD and is trained in providing talk therapy. A

psychiatrist, on the other hand, is a medical doctor
with specialized training in mental health and is

able to prescribe medication. A licensed clinical social worker or licensed professional counselor may also provide talk therapy but may not have the same level of training as a psychologist or psychiatrist.

It is also important to consider whether you are looking for individual therapy, group therapy, or a combination of both. Individual therapy is a one-on-one session with a therapist, while group therapy involves meeting with a group of people who are also struggling with similar issues. Group therapy can be beneficial for those who feel more comfortable sharing their experiences with others and who find support in the group setting.

Another important aspect of finding the right help understands your insurance coverage and whether the therapist or facility you are considering is in-network. This can be a confusing and overwhelming process, but there are resources available such as the National Alliance on Mental Illness (NAMI) that can help guide you through it.

Finally, it is important to remember that finding the right help is not a one-time event, but rather a journey. It may take some time to find the right therapist or treatment plan, and it is okay to switch therapists or try different types of treatment if something isn't working.

One real-life example is Sarah, a mother of two who is struggling with postpartum depression. She initially started seeing a licensed clinical social worker but found that she needed more support than talk therapy alone. She then switched to seeing a psychiatrist who was able to provide medication in addition to therapy, which greatly improved her symptoms.

It is important to remember that seeking help is a courageous step toward improving your mental health. With the right information and resources, you can find the right help and take control of your mental health journey.

Coping Strategies and Support for Mental Health Issues

Living with a mental health condition can be challenging, but there are many coping strategies and support options available that can help individuals manage their symptoms and improve their overall well-being. In this chapter, we will explore different coping strategies and support options for mental health issues, including self-care, therapy, and medication. We will also examine how to access and navigate the mental health care system, and how to find the right support for you.

Self-Care: Self-care is an essential component of managing mental health issues. Self-care strategies can include activities such as exercise, meditation, journaling, and spending time outdoors. For example, exercise has been shown to improve mood, reduce anxiety and depression, and improve overall well-being.

An example of this is Sarah, who has been dealing with depression. She has found that going for a daily walk and practicing yoga has greatly improved her mood and helped her to feel more in control of her symptoms.

Therapy: Therapy, also known as counseling or talk therapy, can be an effective way to manage mental health issues. Different types of therapy, such as cognitive behavioral therapy (CBT) and psychoanalytic therapy can help individuals understand and manage their thoughts, emotions, and behaviors. An example of this is Michael, who has been struggling with anxiety. He has found that cognitive behavioral therapy (CBT) has been very helpful in teaching him how to identify and change negative thought patterns that contribute to his anxiety.

Medication: Medication, such as antidepressants and anti-anxiety medication can also be an effective way to manage mental health issues. Medication can be used alone or in combination with therapy. It is important to work closely with a healthcare professional to find the right medication and dosage for you. An example of this is Rachel, who has been struggling with bipolar disorder. She has found that taking lithium has greatly improved her mood and helped her to manage her symptoms.

Accessing and Navigating the Mental Health Care System: Accessing and navigating the mental health care system can be overwhelming, but it is important to find the right support for you. This can include finding a therapist or counselor, getting a referral to a specialist, and learning about insurance coverage for mental health services. An example of this is Thomas, who has been struggling with addiction. He has found that seeking professional help and going through rehab has been the most effective way for him to manage his addiction.

Finding the Right Support: Finding the right support can be difficult, but it is important to find the right support for you. This can include support groups, peer support, and online resources.

An example of this is Lisa, who has been struggling with PTSD. She has found that joining a support group for individuals with PTSD has been very helpful in providing her with a sense of community and understanding. In summary, chapter 5 will provide a detailed overview of coping strategies and support options for mental health issues, including self-care, therapy, medication, accessing and navigating the mental health care system, and finding the right support. The chapter will also provide real-life examples to help readers understand how these strategies and options may be used in different situations and how they can benefit individuals. The goal of this chapter is to provide readers with a comprehensive understanding of the various support options available to them and to empower them to take control of their mental health and improve their overall well-being.

Chapter 6

THE IMPORTANCE OF SELF-CARE AND MINDFULNESS

Self-care and mindfulness are crucial components of maintaining and improving mental health. This chapter will explore the importance of self-care and mindfulness, with a focus on real-life examples and an entertaining tone.

Self-care is the practice of taking care of oneself in a way that promotes physical, emotional, and mental well-being. It can include things such as getting enough sleep, eating a balanced diet, exercising, and engaging in hobbies that bring joy. For example, Jane, a stay-at-home mom, found that taking a bubble bath and reading a book helped her relax after a long day of taking care of her children.

Mindfulness is the practice of being present and engaged in the current moment, without judgment. Mindfulness can be practiced through meditation, yoga, and other forms of exercise. Research has shown that mindfulness can reduce symptoms of anxiety and depression, and improve overall well-being. For example, Michael, a business executive, found that mindfulness meditation helped him manage the stress of his high-pressure job.

It's important to note that self-care and mindfulness are not one-time solutions, but rather ongoing practices that require consistent effort and commitment. It's important to make self-care and mindfulness a part of your daily routine and to experiment with different strategies to see what works best for you. It's also important to remember that self-care and mindfulness are not just about self-indulgence, but they're also about self-preservation. They're about taking care of oneself in a way that will help keep you healthy and strong, physically, emotionally, and mentally. It's also important to remember that self-care and mindfulness are not just about self-indulgence, but they're also about self-preservation. They're about taking care of oneself in a way that will help keep you healthy and strong, physically, emotionally, and mentally.

In summary, this chapter has provided an overview of the importance of self-care and mindfulness in maintaining and improving mental health. Incorporating these practices into your daily routine can help you manage symptoms of mental health conditions and improve overall well-being. Remember to be kind to yourself, give yourself time and space, and experiment with different strategies to find what works best for you.

Coping Strategies and Self-Care for Mental Health

Mental health conditions can be overwhelming and difficult to manage, but there are coping strategies and self-care practices that can help. This chapter will explore different coping strategies and self-care practices, with a focus on real-life examples and an entertaining tone. One important coping strategy is mindfulness. Mindfulness is the practice of being present and engaged in the current moment, without judgment. Mindfulness can be practiced through meditation, yoga, and other forms of exercise. Research has shown that mindfulness can reduce symptoms of anxiety and depression, and improve overall well-being.

Another coping strategy is journaling. Writing down your thoughts and feelings can be a powerful tool for understanding and managing them. Journaling can also help you identify patterns and triggers, and can serve as a record of your progress over time. Self-care practices are also important for managing mental health. Self-care includes activities that promote physical, emotional and mental well-being. It can include things such as getting enough sleep, eating a balanced diet, exercising, and engaging in hobbies that bring joy. For example, John, a college student who struggles with anxiety, found that taking a walk outside and listening to music helped to reduce his symptoms. He also started journaling as a way to process his thoughts and feelings. It's also important to remember that self-care is not just about self-indulgence, but it's also about self-preservation. It's about taking care of oneself in a way that will help keep you healthy and strong, physically, emotionally, and mentally. It's also important to remember that self-care is not just about self-indulgence, but it's also about self-preservation. It's about taking care of oneself in a way that will help keep you healthy and strong, physically, emotionally, and mentally. It is important to remember that everyone's needs are different and it's important to find what works for you. There's no one size fits all approach to self-care, and it's important to experiment with different strategies to see what works for you. In summary, this chapter has provided an overview of various coping strategies and self-care practices that can help manage mental health conditions. These strategies and practices can be used in combination with therapy and medication to create a comprehensive approach to managing mental health. Remember to be kind to yourself and give yourself the time and space to try different strategies and find what works best for you.

Chapter 7

POSITIVE THINKING AND COPING STRATEGIES

Positive thinking and coping strategies are essential tools for managing mental health conditions and promoting well-being. This chapter will explore the benefits of positive thinking and various coping strategies, using real-life examples, illustrations, and citations to research studies.

Positive thinking is the practice of focusing on the good in situations, rather than dwelling on the negative. Research has shown that positive thinking can lead to several benefits, including improved mood, reduced stress, and better physical health. Some examples of positive thinking techniques include:

Reframing negative thoughts: Instead of focusing on the negative aspects of a situation, try to find the positive. For example, instead of thinking "I'll never be able to finish this project," try thinking "I may not know how to finish this project yet, but I'll figure it out."

Practicing gratitude: Take time each day to think about things you're grateful for. This can be as simple as writing down a few things you're thankful for in a journal or sharing your gratitude with someone else.

Engaging in positive self-talk: Be kind to yourself and talk to yourself the way you would talk to a friend. Instead of criticizing yourself for making a mistake, try to remind yourself that everyone makes mistakes and that you can learn from them.

Coping strategies are specific techniques or behaviors used to manage stress and other negative emotions. Some examples of coping strategies include:

Exercise: Regular physical activity has been shown to have a positive impact on mental health, reducing stress and improving mood.

Journaling: Writing about your thoughts and feelings can help you process them and gain insight.

Relaxation techniques: Mindfulness, deep breathing, and progressive muscle relaxation are all effective ways to reduce stress and promote relaxation.

Social support: Talking to friends and family about your feelings can provide support and help you feel less alone.

It's important to note that not all coping strategies work for everyone, so it's essential to experiment and find what works best for you. Additionally, it's important to speak with a qualified mental health professional before trying any coping strategies to ensure they are appropriate and safe for you.

In this chapter, we will also explore different case studies, with illustrations that show how positive thinking and coping strategies have helped real people manage their mental health conditions. We will also provide citations to research studies that support the effectiveness of these techniques. By the end of this chapter, readers will have a better understanding of the benefits of positive thinking and coping strategies, and feel empowered to incorporate them into their own lives.

Chapter 8

THERAPY AND MEDICATION:
TREATMENT OPTIONS FOR MENTAL HEALTH

Mental health treatment can be a challenging and overwhelming process, especially for those who are new to the experience. In this chapter, we will explore the different therapy and medication options available for treating mental health conditions. When it comes to treating mental health conditions, there are a variety of options available. Some individuals may find relief through therapy alone, while others may require a combination of therapy and medication. In this chapter, we will explore the different types of therapy and medication available for treating mental health conditions, as well as their benefits and potential drawbacks

First, let's discuss therapy. Several types of therapy can be effective in treating mental health conditions, including cognitive-behavioral therapy (CBT), dialectical behavior therapy (DBT), and psychodynamic therapy. Each of these therapies has its unique approach and can be tailored to the individual needs of the patient.

Cognitive-behavioral therapy (CBT) is a form of talk therapy that focuses on the relationship between thoughts, feelings, and behaviors. The goal of CBT is to identify and change negative patterns of thought and behavior that can contribute to mental health conditions. Studies have shown that CBT is effective in treating conditions such as depression, anxiety, and post-traumatic stress disorder (PTSD).

One of the most common types of therapy for mental health conditions is cognitive-behavioral therapy (CBT). CBT is a form of talk therapy that focuses on helping individuals change negative patterns of thought and behavior. This type of therapy is effective in treating a variety of conditions, including depression, anxiety, and post-traumatic stress disorder (PTSD) (American Psychological Association, 2020).

Another type of therapy that is often used to treat mental health conditions is interpersonal therapy (IPT). IPT is a form of talk therapy that focuses on improving communication and relationships with others. This type of therapy is effective in treating conditions such as depression and anxiety (American Psychological Association, 2020).

Dialectical behavior therapy (DBT) is a type of CBT that is specifically designed for individuals with borderline personality disorder (BPD). DBT aims to help individuals regulate their emotions, improve relationships, and reduce self-destructive behaviors.

Psychodynamic therapy is a form of talk therapy that is based on the idea that early life experiences can shape a person's thoughts, feelings, and behaviors. The goal of psychodynamic therapy is to help individuals understand and resolve unconscious conflicts that may be contributing to their mental health condition. In addition to therapy, medication can also be an effective treatment option for mental health conditions. Several classes of medication are commonly used to treat mental health conditions, including antidepressants, antipsychotics, and mood stabilizers.

Antidepressants, such as selective serotonin reuptake inhibitors (SSRIs) and tricyclic antidepressants, are commonly used to treat depression, anxiety, and obsessive-compulsive disorder (OCD). Antipsychotics, such as risperidone and olanzapine, are often used to treat schizophrenia and bipolar disorder. Mood stabilizers, such as lithium and valproic acid, are used to treat bipolar disorder.

It's important to note that finding the right treatment can take time and may involve trying different therapy and medication options. It's also important to work with a mental health professional who can help you navigate the treatment process.

In conclusion, therapy and medication are important options for treating mental health conditions. It's important to work with a mental health professional to find the right treatment plan for you. Remember, treatment is a journey and it's okay to take the time you need to find the right fit for you.

Chapter 9

ALTERNATIVE THERAPIES FOR MENTAL HEALTH

In addition to traditional therapy and medication, there are a variety of alternative therapies that can be effective in treating mental health conditions. These therapies may include practices such as yoga, meditation, acupuncture, and herbal medicine. Yoga and meditation are effective in reducing symptoms of anxiety and depression. Yoga, in particular, has been found to improve overall well-being and reduce stress. A study conducted by the International Journal of Yoga found that regular yoga practice led to a decrease in symptoms of depression, anxiety, and stress in participants (Chen, et al, 2017). Acupuncture, a form of traditional Chinese medicine, has also been found to be effective in treating mental health conditions. A review of studies conducted by the Journal of Affective Disorders found that acupuncture was effective in reducing symptoms of depression and anxiety (Xu, et al, 2017).

Herbal medicine, including the use of supplements such as St. John's Wort and omega-3 fatty acids, may also be effective in treating mental health conditions. A study conducted by the Journal of Clinical Psychiatry found that omega-3 supplements were effective in reducing symptoms of depression in adults (Kiecolt-Glaser, et al, 2017). It is important to note that alternative therapies should not be used as a replacement for traditional therapy and medication, but rather as a complement to them. It is also important to consult with a healthcare professional before starting any alternative therapy to ensure that it is safe and appropriate for you.

Chapter 10

BUILDING A SUPPORT NETWORK

Having a strong support network is essential for individuals who are dealing with mental health issues. A support network can provide emotional, practical, and social support, which can play a crucial role in recovery and overall well-being. This chapter will provide an in-depth understanding of how to build a support network, as well as the benefits and importance of having one. One way to build a support network is to connect with others who have similar experiences. This can be done through support groups, therapy groups, or online communities. Being able to connect with others who understand what you are going through can provide a sense of validation, understanding, and encouragement. Another way to build a support network is to seek out professional help. This can include talking to a therapist, counselor, or psychiatrist.

These professionals can provide guidance and support, as well as offer different treatment options, such as therapy and medication. It's also important to have a support network made up of family and friends. They can provide practical support, such as helping with tasks or errands, and emotional support, such as being a listening ear. It's important to have open and honest communication with your loved ones about your mental health, so they can understand and support you in the best way possible.

In addition to these support options, it's also important to take care of yourself. This includes engaging in self-care practices such as exercise, healthy eating, and getting enough sleep. Mindfulness practices like yoga, meditation, and journaling can also be beneficial in building a support network. It's important to remember that building a support network takes time and effort, but it can make a significant difference in your mental health journey. With the right support and resources, individuals can learn to manage their mental health conditions and lead fulfilling lives.

It is important to understand that mental health is a journey and it is not something that can be fixed overnight. Building a support network is essential in managing and improving mental health.

A support network can consist of family, friends, healthcare professionals, support groups, and other resources.

Reach out to family and friends: Share your struggles with loved ones who you trust and who will be there to support you. They can provide emotional support and help you navigate through difficult times.

Join a support group: Support groups can be a great way to connect with others who are going through similar experiences. They provide a safe and non-judgmental environment where individuals can share their struggles and provide support to one another.

Find a therapist: A therapist can provide professional support and guidance. They can help you work through your emotions and develop coping mechanisms to manage your mental health.

Connect with online communities: The internet has made it easier than ever to connect with others who understand what you are going through. Online communities such as forums and social media groups can provide support and resources for those struggling with mental health issues.

Volunteer: Volunteering can be a great way to give back to the community and also provides a sense of purpose and fulfillment. It can also be a great way to meet new people and build a support network.

Utilize Employee Assistance Programs (EAP): Many workplaces offer Employee Assistance Programs (EAP) that provide employees with confidential counseling, resources, and support.

Contact a crisis hotline: Crisis hotlines are available 24/7 and provide support for individuals in crisis. These hotlines can provide immediate help and connect individuals with resources for ongoing support.

Practice self-care: Self-care is essential in building a support network. Engage in activities that make you feel good, such as exercise, meditation, and spending time with loved ones.

Be open to new experiences: try new things and meet new people, it can open up opportunities for new friendships and support.

Remember that it's okay to ask for help: Asking for help is not a sign of weakness. It takes courage to admit that you need support and it is an important step in building a support network.

It's important to remember that building a support network takes time and effort, but it is worth it in the long run. Your support network can provide you with the resources and emotional support you need to manage your mental health. Always remember to treat yourself with kindness and compassion, and never hesitate to reach out for help.

Chapter 11

HOW TO TALK ABOUT MENTAL HEALTH

Mental health is a topic that affects everyone, yet it is often stigmatized and misunderstood. In this chapter, we will explore the importance of open and honest communication when it comes to discussing mental health and how we can break down the barriers that prevent people from seeking help.

First, it is essential to understand the importance of language when talking about mental health. The words we use can have a significant impact on how people view and understand mental illness. For example, using terms like "crazy" or "psycho" to describe someone with a mental health condition can perpetuate negative stereotypes and make it harder for that person to seek help. Instead, it is essential to use person-first language, such as "a person living with depression" rather than "a depressed person."

Another important aspect of discussing mental health is being aware of the various cultural and societal factors that can affect how people view and talk about mental illness. For example, in some cultures, mental health is not talked about openly, and people may feel ashamed or embarrassed to seek help. It is essential to be mindful of these cultural differences and to approach the topic of mental health with sensitivity and understanding. Another key aspect of talking about mental health is providing accurate and reliable information. This includes understanding the different types of mental health conditions, the causes, symptoms, and treatments available. This can help to reduce the stigma associated with mental health and make it easier for people to seek help. In addition, it is essential to be an active listener when someone is sharing their experiences with mental health. This means showing empathy, providing a safe and non-judgmental space for them to talk, and being there to support them through the process.

Lastly, it is important to know when and how to seek professional help. This includes understanding the different types of therapy and medication available and knowing when it is necessary to seek out a mental health professional.

In conclusion, talking about mental health is essential for breaking down the barriers that prevent people from seeking help. By using appropriate language, being mindful of cultural differences, providing accurate information, being an active listener, and knowing when and how to seek professional help, we can create a more open and understanding society where people can feel comfortable discussing their mental health.

Chapter 12

ADVOCATING FOR MENTAL HEALTH IN YOUR COMMUNITY

Mental health advocacy is the act of working to improve the overall well-being of individuals and communities affected by mental health conditions. It involves raising awareness, educating the public, and fighting for policies and systems that support mental health and well-being. In this chapter, we will explore ways in which you can advocate for mental health in your community.

Advocacy is the act of speaking out and working to promote a particular cause or issue. In the context of mental health, advocacy means working to improve the lives of those living with mental health conditions, as well as raising awareness and understanding about mental health in general. Advocacy can take many forms, from individual actions to larger social movements.

First, it is important to understand the importance of mental health advocacy. Mental health conditions are prevalent in our society, affecting one in five adults in the United States alone. Despite this, mental health often receives less attention and resources than physical health.

By advocating for mental health, we can work towards a society where mental health is valued and supported in the same way as physical health.

A way to advocate for mental health in your community is through education and awareness. This can be done through organizing or participating in events such as mental health fairs, workshops, or seminars. These events provide a platform for individuals and organizations to share information and resources about mental health, and can also help to reduce the stigma surrounding mental health conditions.

One important way to advocate for mental health in your community is to educate yourself and others about the facts and realities of mental health conditions. This includes understanding the prevalence of mental health conditions, the different types of mental health conditions, and the available treatments. Additionally, it's crucial to be informed about the barriers and stigma that people with mental health conditions often face.

Another way to advocate for mental health is by participating in grassroots campaigns and lobbying for policy change. This can include writing letters to elected officials, participating in rallies and marches, or joining a mental health advocacy organization. By working together, individuals and organizations can push for policies and systems that support mental health and well-being, such as increased funding for mental health research and services, or the implementation of mental health parity laws. It is also important to advocate for mental health in your personal and professional life.

Another way to advocate for mental health in your community is to use your voice to influence public policy and systems. This can include writing letters, signing petitions, and meeting with elected officials to share your concerns and advocate for mental health-related legislation and policies.

This can include speaking up when you see discrimination or stigma related to mental health or creating a supportive and inclusive environment in your workplace or community.

By taking these actions, we can work towards a society where mental health is treated with the respect and attention it deserves. Ultimately, advocating for mental health in your community means working to create a more supportive and understanding environment for those living with mental health conditions. It means speaking out against discrimination and prejudice and working to promote awareness, understanding, and access to mental health resources and support. It's important to note that advocacy should always be done ethically and professionally and with the consent of the person you're advocating for. It's also important to be aware of any power dynamics that may exist in the situation and to be mindful of those who may be marginalized or disadvantaged.

In conclusion, advocating for mental health in your community is an important way to improve the overall well-being of individuals and communities affected by mental health conditions. Through education and awareness, grassroots campaigns, and personal and professional advocacy, we can work towards a society where mental health is valued and supported.

Advocating for mental health in your community is a crucial step towards creating a more supportive and understanding society for those living with mental health conditions. By educating yourself and others, speaking out against discrimination and stigmatization, supporting local organizations and initiatives, using your voice to influence public policy, and being mindful of ethical considerations, you can make a meaningful impact in your community.

Chapter 13

MAINTAINING GOOD MENTAL HEALTH: TIPS AND STRATEGIES

Maintaining good mental health is an ongoing process that requires a combination of self-care, professional support, and community involvement. In this chapter, we will explore various tips and strategies that can help you maintain your mental well-being.

First, it is important to understand that everyone's needs and experiences are unique. What works for one person may not work for another, so it is important to find what works best for you. Some people find that regular exercise and physical activity are essential for maintaining good mental health, while others find that mindfulness practices like yoga and meditation are more beneficial.

In addition to physical activities, it is important to engage in activities that you enjoy and that bring you a sense of purpose. This can include hobbies, volunteering, or pursuing a creative endeavor. Having a sense of purpose and something to look forward to can help to boost your mood and reduce stress.

An important strategy for maintaining good mental health is to practice self-care. This can include activities such as meditating, journaling, or taking a relaxing bath. It is important to find activities that you enjoy and that help you to relax and de-stress. Additionally, it is important to make time for yourself each day, even if it is just a few minutes, to do something that you enjoy or that makes you feel good.

Another important aspect of maintaining good mental health is establishing and maintaining healthy relationships. This includes connecting with friends and family, as well as seeking out support from professionals such as therapists or counselors. Strong social connections can help to reduce feelings of isolation and loneliness, which can contribute to mental health issues. Another important strategy for maintaining good mental health is to build and maintain positive relationships. This can include connecting with friends and family, joining a club or group, or volunteering in your community. Research has shown that social support is essential for good mental health and that people who have strong social connections tend to be happier and healthier.

It is also important to establish healthy habits and routines. This includes getting enough sleep, eating a balanced diet, and avoiding substance abuse. These habits can help to regulate your mood and reduce stress. Lastly, it is important to be aware of the warning signs of mental health issues and seek help if needed.

This can include talking to a therapist or counselor, joining a support group, or taking medication. Remember, seeking help is not a sign of weakness, but rather an important step toward maintaining good mental health. In summary, maintaining good mental health requires a combination of self-care, professional support, and community involvement. Engaging in activities you enjoy, having a sense of purpose, building and maintaining healthy relationships, establishing healthy habits and routines, and being aware of warning signs are all important steps toward maintaining good mental health.

It is important to seek help if you are struggling with mental health issues. This can include talking to a therapist or counselor, joining a support group, or taking medication. Remember, it is not a sign of weakness to ask for help, and there is no shame in seeking treatment for mental health issues.

In conclusion, maintaining good mental health is essential for leading a happy and fulfilling life. It is important to take care of yourself physically, practice self-care, build and maintain positive relationships, and seek help if you are struggling with mental health issues. Remember, it is possible to maintain good mental health even if you are struggling with mental illness, and it is important to take an active role in your mental health.

Chapter 14

MANAGING STRESS AND FINDING
BALANCE IN YOUR LIFE

Stress is a normal part of life, but when it becomes chronic, it
can have a detrimental effect on our mental and physical
health. In this chapter, we will explore the causes of stress and
the impact it can have on our mental health, as well
as strategies for managing and reducing stress.

One of the main causes of stress is the
feeling of being overwhelmed. This can happen
when we take on too many responsibilities at once,
or when we are faced with unexpected challenges. It
can also be caused by a lack of control over our
environment, or by feeling unsupported by those
around us. When stress becomes chronic, it can lead
to a range of mental health conditions, including
anxiety and depression.

It can also lead to physical health problems, such as heart disease and high blood pressure. To manage stress, it is important to identify the sources of stress in our lives and take steps to reduce or eliminate them. This can include setting boundaries, learning to say no, and delegating tasks to others. Another important strategy for managing stress is to engage in self-care practices. This can include activities such as exercise, meditation, and journaling. These practices can help to reduce the physical and emotional symptoms of stress, and can also help to improve our overall well-being. In addition to managing stress, it is also important to find balance in our lives. This can include making time for hobbies and activities that we enjoy, spending time with loved ones, and getting enough sleep. It is also important to seek support from others. This can include talking to friends and family or seeking professional help from a therapist or counselor.

Stress is a normal part of life, but when it becomes overwhelming, it can take a toll on our mental and physical health. Finding balance and managing stress is essential to maintaining good mental health. In this chapter, we will explore 14 ways to manage stress and find balance in your life.

From mindfulness practices to setting boundaries, these strategies can help you cope with stress and improve your overall well-being.

14 Ways to Managing Stress and Finding Balance in Your Life

Mindfulness: Mindfulness practices such as meditation and yoga can help you focus on the present moment and reduce stress.

Exercise: Regular physical activity can help reduce stress and improve your mood.

Sleep: Adequate sleep is crucial for managing stress and maintaining good mental health.

Nutrition: Eating a healthy diet can help reduce stress and improve your overall well-being.

Time management: Setting realistic goals and managing your time effectively can help reduce stress.

Boundaries: Setting boundaries with work, friends, and family can help you balance your time and reduce stress.

Support network: Having a strong support network of friends and family can help you cope with stress.

Humor: Laughing and finding humor in everyday life can help reduce stress and improve your mood.

Relaxation techniques: Relaxation techniques such as deep breathing and progressive muscle relaxation can help you reduce stress.

Creativity: Engaging in creative activities such as art, music, and writing can help you cope with stress and improve your overall well-being.

Spirituality: Connecting with your spirituality can help you find meaning and purpose in life, which can reduce stress.

Nature: Spending time in nature can help reduce stress and improve your mood.

Gratitude: Practicing gratitude can help you focus on the positive aspects of your life and reduce stress.

Therapy: Talking to a therapist can help you work through stress and develop coping strategies.

Finally, managing stress and finding balance in your life is essential to maintaining good mental health. By incorporating these 14 strategies into your daily routine, you can reduce stress and improve your overall well-being. Remember to be kind to yourself and seek help when needed. It's important to remember that everyone experiences stress differently, so finding the right stress management technique for you may take some experimentation. Consult with a mental health professional if you need additional support.

Chapter 15

THE IMPACT OF SOCIAL DETERMINANTS OF HEALTH ON MENTAL HEALTH

Mental health is a complex and multifaceted issue, and many factors can contribute to its development and maintenance.
One of the most important factors to consider when examining mental health is the impact of social determinants of health. Social determinants of health are the conditions in which people are born, grow, live, work, and age that can have a profound impact on their health and well-being.

As we explore how social determinants of health can affect mental health and the strategies that can be used to mitigate these effects. We will begin by defining the various social determinants of health and their impact on mental health.

Socioeconomic status, for example, has a significant impact on mental health. People living in poverty are more likely to experience mental health issues than those with higher incomes. This is due to some factors, including lack of access to resources, lack of social support, and exposure to stressful life events.

Education is another important social determinant of health that can affect mental health. People with higher levels of education are more likely to have better mental health outcomes than those with lower levels of education. This is due in part to the fact that people with higher levels of education are more likely to have access to resources, social support, and opportunities for personal growth and development.

In addition to socioeconomic status and education, other social determinants of health that can affect mental health include race and ethnicity, gender, sexual orientation, and geographic location. For example, people of color and those in rural areas are more likely to experience mental health disparities than those in more affluent areas. To address these disparities, it is important to take a holistic approach to mental health that incorporates a wide range of interventions, including access to resources, social support, and opportunities for personal growth and development. This may include things like community-based programs, peer support groups, and mental health promotion and prevention initiatives.

In addition, it is important to recognize that mental health is not just an individual issue, but rather a societal issue that requires a collective effort to address. This means that policymakers, community leaders, and other stakeholders must work together to create a culture of support for mental health and to promote policies and programs that address the social determinants of health.

In conclusion, this chapter has highlighted the important role that social determinants of health play in mental health, and the strategies that can be used to mitigate their impact. By understanding how social determinants of health can affect mental health, we can work to create a more equitable and supportive society for all.

Chapter 16

THE IMPACT OF SOCIAL DETERMINANTS OF HEALTH ON MENTAL HEALTH

It is well established that physical and mental health are interconnected. The state of one's physical health can have a significant impact on their mental well-being, and vice versa. This chapter will explore the connection between physical and mental health, and how they can affect one another. One of the key ways in which physical health can impact mental health is through chronic illnesses. Conditions such as heart disease, diabetes, and cancer can take a toll on an individual's emotional and psychological well-being. Studies have shown that people with chronic illnesses are at a higher risk for developing mental health conditions such as depression and anxiety. In addition, physical illnesses can also exacerbate existing mental health conditions.

For example, individuals with chronic pain may experience increased levels of anxiety and depression. This is because chronic pain can make it difficult for individuals to engage in daily activities, which can lead to feelings of hopelessness and despair. On the other hand, mental health conditions can also have a significant impact on physical health. For example, individuals with depression are at a higher risk for developing heart disease and other cardiovascular conditions. This is because depression can lead to unhealthy lifestyle choices, such as smoking, overeating, and lack of physical activity. Another example is an anxiety disorder, it can manifest itself in physical symptoms such as headaches, muscle tension, and fatigue. These physical symptoms can further contribute to feelings of anxiety and a lack of well-being. It is important to note that the connection between physical and mental health is not always straightforward. There can be multiple factors at play, and it is often difficult to determine the exact cause-and-effect relationship. However, one thing is certain: addressing both physical and mental health is crucial for overall well-being. There are several ways in which individuals can work to improve both their physical and mental health.

One of the most effective ways is through exercise. Regular physical activity has been shown to have a positive impact on both physical and mental health. Exercise can improve cardiovascular health, help with weight management, and reduce stress and anxiety. Another important strategy is to maintain a healthy diet. Eating a well-balanced diet that is rich in fruits, vegetables, and whole grains can help to improve physical health and reduce the risk of chronic illness. Lastly, it is important to seek help when needed. If an individual is experiencing symptoms of a mental health condition or chronic illness, it is important to seek professional help. This can include seeing a doctor, therapist, or another mental health professional. With the right treatment and support, individuals can work to improve both their physical and mental health.

Global Mental Health: Understanding and Addressing Mental Health Disparities and Inequalities

Mental health is a global issue that affects individuals from all walks of life, regardless of race, ethnicity, or socioeconomic status. However, certain populations are more vulnerable to mental health disparities and inequalities than others.

First, it is important to understand that mental health is not just the absence of mental illness, but also encompasses an individual's overall well-being and ability to function in their daily life. This includes factors such as emotional, psychological, and social well-being. One of the key contributors to mental health disparities and inequalities in social determinants of health. Social determinants of health refer to the various social, economic, and environmental factors that influence an individual's health and well-being. Examples of social determinants of health include poverty, education, employment, and access to healthcare. These factors can have a significant impact on an individual's mental health, with individuals from marginalized communities often experiencing worse mental health outcomes. Another important factor to consider is the cultural context in which mental health is understood and addressed. Mental health stigma, cultural beliefs and values, and the availability of mental health services can vary greatly between cultures. This can lead to disparities in access to mental health care and treatment, as well as in the way mental health is perceived and discussed. To address global mental health disparities and inequalities, it is important to take a holistic approach that addresses both individual and structural factors.

This includes increasing access to mental health services and resources for marginalized communities, addressing social determinants of health, and working to reduce mental health stigma and discrimination. It is also important to collaborate with community-based organizations and local partners to understand and address the specific needs and cultural contexts of different communities. This includes working with traditional healers and incorporating traditional healing practices into mental health care. In addition, global mental health initiatives must prioritize the voices and perspectives of marginalized communities, including those from low-income countries, to truly address and address the root causes of mental health disparities and inequalities. Examples of such initiatives include the World Health Organization's Mental Health Action Plan 2013-2020, which aims to improve access to mental health care and reduce the stigma surrounding mental illness, and the Mental Health Innovation Network, which brings together organizations and individuals working to improve mental health globally. By understanding and addressing the various factors that contribute to global mental health disparities and inequalities, we can work towards a world where all individuals have the opportunity to achieve optimal mental health and well-being.

In conclusion, the connection between physical and mental health is complex and multifaceted. It is important to recognize that physical and mental health is interdependent, and addressing both is crucial for overall well-being. By implementing strategies such as exercise, healthy eating, and seeking professional help when needed, individuals can work to improve both their physical and mental health.

Chapter 17

MENTAL HEALTH IN DIFFERENT CULTURAL CONTEXTS

Mental health is an important topic that affects people from all walks of life and cultures. However, how mental health is perceived, understood, and treated can vary greatly depending on the cultural context. In this chapter, we will explore how different cultures view and approach mental health, as well as how biblical teachings can guide us in understanding and addressing mental health in a culturally sensitive way.

It's important to note that in many cultures, mental health is not always viewed as a separate entity from physical health. In some Eastern cultures, for example, the mind and body are seen as interconnected and mental health is often treated through holistic practices such as acupuncture, yoga, and meditation. In contrast, Western cultures tend to view mental health as separate from physical health, and often rely on medication and talk therapy as the primary treatment options.

Mental health is a global issue that affects people of all cultures and backgrounds. However, the prevalence and presentation of mental health issues can vary widely across different cultures. It is important to take into account cultural context when addressing mental health, as cultural beliefs and practices can have a significant impact on an individual's mental well-being.

In the United States, for example, anxiety and depression are among the most commonly reported mental health issues. According to the National Institute of Mental Health, 18.1% of adults in the U.S. experience anxiety disorder, and 7.6% experience depression.

In China, mental health is a relatively new concept and there are still a lot of stigmas associated with it. However, the rate of mental health issues is increasing in China, with depression and anxiety being the most commonly reported.

In Africa, mental health issues are often stigmatized and not well understood. Many people with mental health issues in Africa do not receive appropriate treatment or support, and traditional healing practices are often relied upon instead.

In the United Kingdom, the rate of mental health issues is relatively high, with 1 in 4 people experiencing a mental health problem each year. The most common mental health issues in the UK are anxiety and depression.

It is important to note that the mental health issues that affect different cultures are not limited to the examples provided above. The statistics are likely to vary by country, region, and culture.

However, the Bible teaches that our physical and mental well-being are interconnected, with verses such as Proverbs 17:22 stating, "A cheerful heart is a good medicine, but a crushed spirit dries up the bones." This highlights the importance of taking care of both our physical and mental health to truly be well. Additionally, many cultures have traditional healing practices that are rooted in their religious beliefs. For example, some indigenous cultures believe in the power of spiritual ceremonies and rituals to heal mental health issues. Similarly, Christians may turn to prayer and Bible study as a way to find peace and healing for their mental health struggles.

In the Bible, verses such as Isaiah 41:10 "So do not fear, for I am with you; do not be dismayed, for I am your God. I will strengthen you and help you; I will uphold you with my righteous right hand" and Psalm 34:18 "The Lord is close to the brokenhearted and saves those who are crushed in spirit." These verses provide comfort and remind us that God is always with us, providing strength and support during difficult times. Additionally, Proverbs 17:22 says "A cheerful heart is a good medicine, but a crushed spirit dries up the bones." This verse highlights the importance of maintaining a positive attitude and looking after our emotional well-being.

One important aspect of understanding and addressing mental health in different cultural contexts is recognizing and valuing the unique strengths and coping mechanisms that each culture brings. For example, research has shown that people from collectivistic cultures, such as many Asian cultures, often find strength and support in their community and family, while people from individualistic cultures, such as many Western cultures, may prioritize self-reliance and independence.

Furthermore, there are cultural and religious stigmas that can prevent individuals from seeking help for their mental health issues. It is important to educate and raise awareness about the importance of mental health and the available resources in a culturally sensitive manner. Ultimately, it is important to approach mental health in different cultural contexts with empathy, understanding, and a willingness to learn. As Proverbs 3:5-6 states, "Trust in the Lord with all your heart and lean not on your understanding; in all your ways submit to him, and he will make your paths straight." By following this guidance and seeking to understand and support one another, we can work towards building a more inclusive and supportive community for all.

It is important for all individuals to be culturally sensitive and aware, and to work with mental health professionals who are culturally competent. This will help to ensure that individuals receive the most appropriate and effective treatment for their mental health needs.

Chapter 18

Conclusion: Empowering Yourself to Take Control of Your Mental Health

Mental health is a crucial aspect of overall well-being, and it is essential to understand the various factors that contribute to it. In this chapter, we have explored the causes and triggers of mental health issues, the importance of self-care and mindfulness, positive thinking and coping strategies, therapy and medication, alternative therapies, building a support network, how to talk about mental health, advocating for mental health in your community, maintaining good mental health, managing stress, and the impact of social determinants of health on mental health. Additionally, we have examined the connection between physical and mental health, as well as the cultural context of mental health. One of the most significant takeaways from this chapter is the importance of empowerment.

Empowerment means taking control of your mental health, and this can be achieved through various means. For example, understanding the causes and triggers of mental health issues can help you identify potential warning signs and take proactive steps to address them. Additionally, practicing self-care and mindfulness can help you better manage stress and find balance in your life. Positive thinking and coping strategies can also be beneficial in helping you navigate difficult situations and manage negative thoughts and emotions. Another key aspect of empowerment is building a support network. Having a support network in place can provide you with the emotional and practical support you need to manage mental health issues. This can include family, friends, and professionals, such as therapists and counselors. Additionally, it is important to be aware of the resources available to you, such as therapy and medication, as well as alternative therapies, such as yoga and meditation. When it comes to advocating for mental health in your community, it is essential to understand the role of social determinants of health.

Social determinants of health refer to the various factors that influence health outcomes, such as income, education, and access to healthcare. By understanding these factors, you can better advocate for policies and programs that promote mental health and well-being. Furthermore, it is important to understand the cultural context of mental health. Different cultures may have different beliefs and attitudes toward mental health, and this can affect how mental health issues are addressed and treated. It is crucial to be sensitive to these cultural differences and to work towards creating a more inclusive and culturally-competent mental health system.

In conclusion, mental health is a complex and multi-faceted issue, and it is essential to take a holistic approach to understand and addressing it. By empowering yourself to take control of your mental health, you can better navigate the mental health system and find the help you need. Additionally, by understanding the various factors that influence mental health, you can advocate for policies and programs that promote mental health and well-being in your community. Remember, it is always important to seek professional help if you are struggling with your mental health, and don't be afraid to reach out for support from loved ones and professionals.

"The Lord is close to the brokenhearted and saves those who are crushed in spirit." - Psalm 34:18 "Come to me, all you who are weary and burdened, and I will give you rest." - Matthew 11:28 "So do not fear, for I am with you; do not be dismayed, for I am your God. I will strengthen you and help you; I will uphold you with my righteous right hand." - Isaiah 41:10

Chapter 19

APPENDIX

These worksheets and exercises are designed to help readers take an active role in their mental health journey and to empower them to take control of their well-being.

1. Mindfulness Worksheet: This worksheet is designed to help readers practice mindfulness, a technique that involves paying attention to the present moment without judgment. It includes exercises such as deep breathing, body scan, and guided imagery.

2. Positive Thinking Worksheet: This worksheet is designed to help readers practice positive thinking, which involves focusing on the good in any situation. It includes exercises such as gratitude journaling and identifying negative thoughts and reframing them into positive thoughts.

3. Coping Strategies Worksheet: This worksheet is designed to help readers identify and practice coping strategies that work for them. It includes exercises

4. such as identifying triggers, brainstorming coping strategies, and evaluating the effectiveness of different coping strategies.

5. Self-Care Plan: This worksheet is designed to help readers create a self-care plan that is tailored to their needs. It includes exercises such as identifying self-care activities, setting self-care goals, and creating a self-care schedule.

6. Support Network Worksheet: This worksheet is designed to help readers identify and build a support network. It includes exercises such as identifying potential support people, creating a list of support people, and brainstorming ways to maintain and strengthen relationships with supportive people.

7. Mental Health Journal: This journal is designed to help readers track their mental health journey. It includes prompts for reflection on mental health symptoms, triggers, coping strategies, self-care activities, and support systems.

8. Therapeutic Writing: This worksheet includes prompts for therapeutic writing, which is a form of self-expression that can help manage stress and process emotions.

These worksheets and exercises are not intended to be a substitute for professional help, but rather as a complement to it. They are also not intended to be used as diagnostic tools. They are meant to serve as a guide for self-reflection and self-improvement. It is always important to consult with a mental health professional if you have any concerns about your mental health.

b

Chapter 20

Glossary: Mental Health Terminology

A

- Anxiety: A feeling of worry, nervousness, or unease about something with an uncertain outcome. Anxiety can be a normal and often healthy emotion, but it can become overwhelming in some individuals and lead to disorders such as Generalized Anxiety Disorder (GAD) or Panic Disorder.

B

- Behavioral therapy: A form of psychotherapy that focuses on identifying and changing negative patterns of thought and behavior.

- Bipolar disorder: A mental health condition characterized by extreme mood swings, from manic highs to depressive lows.

C

- Cognitive therapy: A form of psychotherapy that focuses on identifying and changing negative patterns of thought to improve emotional regulation and overall mental health.

- Coping mechanisms: Strategies and techniques used to manage stress and difficult emotions.

D

- Depression: A mental health condition characterized by persistent feelings of sadness, hopelessness, and a lack of interest in activities.

E

- Empathy: The ability to understand and share the feelings of another person.

- Emotional regulation: The ability to manage and control one's emotions healthily and adaptively.

F

- Family therapy: A form of psychotherapy that involves the whole family in the treatment process.

G

- Generalized Anxiety Disorder (GAD): A disorder characterized by excessive and unrealistic worry about everyday events and activities.

H

- Hypnotherapy: A form of therapy that uses hypnosis to help individuals overcome problems such as phobias, anxiety, and addictions.

I

- Insight therapy: A form of psychotherapy that focuses on helping individuals gain insight into their thoughts, feelings, and behaviors.

M

- Medication: A form of treatment for mental health conditions that involve the use of drugs to alleviate symptoms.

P

- Panic disorder: A disorder characterized by recurrent and unexpected panic attacks, often accompanied by physical symptoms such as heart palpitations, sweating, and trembling.
- Post-traumatic stress disorder (PTSD): A disorder that can develop after a traumatic event, such as a natural disaster, accident, or combat experience. Symptoms include flashbacks, nightmares, and emotional numbing.

S

- Self-care: The practice of taking care of one's physical, emotional, and mental well-being.

- Support group: A group of individuals who share a common problem or concern and meet to provide mutual support and understanding.

T

- Therapy: A form of treatment for mental health conditions that involves talking to a trained mental health professional.

W

- Wellness: A state of overall health and well-being that encompasses physical, emotional, and mental well-being.

Y

- Yoga: A form of exercise that combines physical postures, breathing exercises, and meditation, intending to improve overall health and well-being.

References

Chen, K.C., Chen, P.Y., & Kao, Y.F. (2017). The Effect of Yoga on Depression, Anxiety, and Stress. International Journal of Yoga, 10(1), 11-17. Xu, X., et al. (2017). Acupuncture for Depression: A Systematic Review and Meta-Analysis. Journal of Affective Disorders, 207, 1-10. Kiecolt-Glaser, J.K., et al. (2017). Omega-3 Supplementation Lowers Inflammation and Anxiety in Medical Students: A Randomized Controlled Trial. Journal of Clinical Psychiatry, 78(9), 1340-13

World Health Organization (WHO). (2020). Mental Health. Retrieved from https://www.who.int/health-topics/mental-health/ National Institute of Mental Health (NIMH). (2020). Mental Health Basics

American Psychological Association. (2020). Types of Therapy. Retrieved from https://www.apa.org/topics/therapy/types

National Institute of Mental Health. (2020). Medications for Mental Illnesses. Retrieved from https://www.nimh.nih.gov/health/topics/mental - health-medications/index.shtml

National Institute of Mental Health. (2019). Depression. Retrieved from https://www.nimh.nih.gov/health/topics/depression/index.shtml

National Institute of Mental Health. (2019). Anxiety disorders. Retrieved from https://www.nimh.nih.gov/health/topics/anxiety-disorders/index.shtml

National Institute of Mental Health. (2019). Schizophrenia. Retrieved from https://www.nimh.nih.gov/health/topics/schizophrenia/index.shtml

National Institute of Mental Health. (2019). Bipolar disorder. Retrieved from https://www.nimh.nih.gov/health/topics/bipolar-disorder/index.shtml